TANSY BRIGGS, DACM

The Key to

POSTPARTUM HEALING

Rest
Nourish
Heal

Plan your postpartum
Protect your health

Copyright © 2020 by Tansy Briggs, DACM
All rights reserved. This book or any portion thereof may not be reproduced or used in any manner whatsoever without the express written permission of the publisher except for the use of brief quotations in a book review.

Publishing Services provided by Paper Raven Books
Printed in the United States of America
First Printing, 2020

Paperback ISBN= 978-1-7340561-4-3
Hardback ISBN= 978-1-7340561-5-0

TABLE OF CONTENTS

Acknowledgements — 1

Introduction
How to use this book — 6

Chapter 1: Prepare
Nutrition for pregnancy — 7
Morning sickness — 10
Foods through the trimesters — 12

Chapter 2: Recover
The fourth trimester — 17
The first 10 days — 19
When to seek medical attention — 24

Chapter 3: Heal
Healing basics — 27
Postpartum resting — 28
Abdominal wrapping — 29
Vaginal births — 31
C-section births — 32
Nipple care — 33
Stretch marks — 33
Pelvic floor recovery — 35
Exercise and losing the "baby weight" — 36

Chapter 4: Nourish

How do you keep your digestion warm? 46

Bone loss in pregnancy and lactation 51

Inflammatory foods affecting healing and breastfeeding 54

Summary: What to Buy and Prepare Before Giving Birth 59

In Closing: A New Beginning 61

Appendix

Key nutrients and foods 63

Nutrient needs through the trimesters 64-65

List of foods and corresponding temperatures 66

Resources 67

ACKNOWLEDGMENTS

As a health care professional and a mother, I have both clinical and personal experience with how important the postpartum period is for women's health. Yet, our Western medical systems and culture often overlook this essential time in women's lives, and more needs to be done to address the postpartum health care gap. Traditions from Asian medicine offer an invaluable resource of information and practice that can be complementary to modern Western medicine. I am not naïve enough to think that Western culture or Western women are all of a sudden going to embrace all the Asian traditions of "Zuò yuè zi" (the resting month) and the principles of postpartum care. But, I am certain that there is a way to bridge the gap and provide Western women with an informational and practical platform to better heal postpartum, no matter what their circumstances may be.

When I was pregnant with my son in my last year of acupuncture and Chinese Medicine school, I absorbed as much information as I could about how to address this most precious and vulnerable time for women and babies. I came across a book written by Zita West, a midwife and acupuncturist in the United Kingdom, called *Acupuncture in Pregnancy and Childbirth*. When I opened the book and started reading, I felt like I had finally found what I had been seeking: the integration of the Western approach to pregnancy, labor, and delivery along with acupuncture treatment. Since then, more and more books, courses, and instructors have come on the scene to grow this incredible field. From Debra Betts's *The Essential Guide to Acupuncture in Pregnancy and Childbirth* to Lia Andrews's *7 Times a Woman* and Claudia Citkovitz's *Acupressure and Acupuncture During Birth*, the quality and quantity of information has grown exponentially in recent years. At the end of this book, you can find a list of helpful resources, including books and websites, that align with the principles discussed here and that can further bolster health for new moms and their babies.

I am grateful for every practitioner and patient who has helped to bring these issues to light and has worked to find the best ways to support health and wellness before, during and after pregnancy. My hope is that, with one woman and one baby at a time, this book will help improve their lives and overall health for years to come. I am especially grateful for Darcy Gist for helping me write this book and for Morgan Gist MacDonald and her team at Paper Raven Books for making all the books I have endeavored to write so much better and for bringing them to fruition. Special thanks to all my friends, patients, and family members who have cheered me on and to my husband, who listens and provides support with an unending well of humor and love.

INTRODUCTION

TO TREAT THE CHILD, TREAT THE MOTHER

As an integrative acupuncture and Chinese Medicine practitioner, I have the privilege of seeing many women through the process of fertility and pregnancy. They see me regularly for acupuncture and herbal treatment where we also discuss nutritional needs, how they are feeling, what to expect at every stage, and any other personal stories that tend to come up during the months they share their lives with me. I do my best to help them prepare for the next stage: having their baby. Once they have their baby, I rarely see them in the clinic unless there is a significant health complication. Often, they lament that they need care but can't figure out a way to juggle all of life's demands and make time for coming into the clinic.

The fourth trimester (yes, there are four!) encompasses the first three months after a full-term pregnancy. Unfortunately, it is also known as the forgotten trimester. Postpartum health is more than a women's issue and is certainly more than losing the "baby weight." It is vastly important not only to the woman herself but also to her baby and her family. How mom heals postpartum can have lasting effects on her health throughout her life. In our modern culture, the concept of being "superwoman" is sold as the standard every woman should strive for: have your baby, lose the pregnancy weight, and resume normal life. This notion goes against thousands of years of experience in Asian medicine and wisdom from plenty of other cultures around the world.

In Asian cultures, postpartum care is a traditional practice that has been passed down from grandmother to mother and mother to daughter for many thousands of years. New mothers are fed and cared for by either a hired professional who specializes in this field (confinement doula) or other female members of the family. For 30 to 40 days after birth, caretakers cook specific foods to support the new mother, massage her with oils, prepare baths of ginger water, and co-care for the babies. Traditional practices like this help the new mothers recover postpartum and prevent premature aging. There are many benefits of this traditional practice focusing on diet, lifestyle, and self-care during this time period.

This all sounds lovely, right? Sadly, these traditions are not generally known or carried out by the average modern Western woman, nor are they promoted through the average Western medical advice or researched in modern studies. (Hopefully, some day we will have more comprehensive data regarding cultural traditions of postpartum care to be used in conventional medicine.) Generally, the mother is seen about six weeks postpartum for a checkup. There is so much healing to be done in these six weeks! So, how can we support proper postpartum healing within the constraints of the average Western lifestyle and expectations?

Proper healing postpartum may help prevent and heal:

- Postpartum depression
- Hormonal imbalances
- Uterine prolapse
- Urinary incontinence
- Diastasis recti
- Weight gain
- Premature aging

- Body aches

- Hemorrhoids

- Injuries and pain

- Imbalances that could lead to other diseases later in life such as thyroid problems, chronic fatigue, osteoporosis, and increased symptoms with perimenopause and menopause

While little research has been conducted to systematically evaluate the effects of acupuncture and Traditional Chinese Medicine on these issues, in my clinical experience of over 20 years of practice treating women of all ages, I have seen the positive results time and time again. I have so many examples of women who have finally been able to come to me for treatment, sometimes months or years after giving birth, and say, "I just haven't felt right since having my baby." Their ailments span a vast range of symptoms and syndromes, including chronic pain, fatigue, insomnia, anxiety, weak immune systems, incontinence, irregular menstrual cycles, and depression, just to name a few.

Since our Western health care system largely ignores postpartum healing, mothers are under pressure to "get on with it." Mothers are told that they should go back to work, lose the baby weight, and care for their new family at home. This can be a lonely, isolating experience for women. It is ironic that many studies have shown that this vulnerable time for women and children is also a very important period of time that can have profound impact for their health affecting the rest of their lives. I don't expect that all of a sudden we will fully adopt the Asian practice of postpartum care, nor do I think those practices would fit Western culture in the same way. But, there are many things we can do to aid and support postpartum healing, even if one is unable to come in for regular care in the clinic or have access to acupuncture and Traditional Chinese Medicine. You will learn a lot of tools in this book to support yourself postpartum, and I encourage you to also seek out professional care, which is even more accessible these days with increased access to telehealth.

■ HOW TO USE THIS BOOK

This book is designed to help you prepare for your pregnancy through all its stages so you can really recover and heal during the fourth trimester and beyond. Where appropriate, it will indicate what you should prepare before having your baby. After you have your baby, there will be sections that may or may not apply to you and your healing process, so you can thumb through and find the topics most relevant to you. If you are coming to this book after having your baby, it is never too late to take active steps for healing.

There are many other wonderful books and resources on healthy pregnancy and how to optimize your baby's health. I encourage you to seek advice from a variety of sources in conjunction with this book and to learn as much as you can to decide what is best for you and your baby.

Please note: The views and nutritional and herbal information expressed in this book are not intended to be a substitute for conventional medical service. If you have or suspect that you have a medical problem, promptly contact your health care provider. Please continue to work with qualified medical professionals as you engage in the information and materials in this book. No information offered here should be interpreted as a diagnosis of any disease, nor an attempt to treat or prevent or cure any disease or condition. Information and statements regarding products and/or services discussed in this book have not been evaluated by the Food and Drug Administration, and products and services are not intended to diagnose, treat, cure, or prevent any disease.

CHAPTER 1: PREPARE

Healing postpartum begins with a healthy pregnancy. Intentional nutrition and lifestyle adjustments can enhance any pregnancy, but how do you know what's best for you, your body, and your baby? Guided by key principles from Traditional Chinese Medicine and the latest research findings, this chapter offers strategies to address commonplace pregnancy-related issues and sets you on the path towards long-term health for you and your baby. Most importantly, consult with your doctor before making any dietary or lifestyle changes discussed in this book during or after your pregnancy.

▪ NUTRITION FOR PREGNANCY

Nutrition during pregnancy shouldn't be dramatically different from your typical diet, since this can create shifts or imbalances that might affect your pregnancy. Incorporate changes slowly and follow your own intuition about food, which is heightened during this time. You should expect to gain about 3 or 4 pounds per month throughout your first three trimesters, about 30 to 35 pounds total. Weight gain is a normal and healthy part of your pregnancy!

▪ Protein

Protein serves as an essential and, in my clinical experience, an undervalued nutrient source that helps protect the health of you and your baby. Sometimes it might feel like a job to intentionally eat this much protein, but the benefits are worth it. You will experience less nausea, a stronger pregnancy, fewer blood sugar fluctuations, and healthy weight gain. Protein supports healthy tissues, muscles, and blood supply and proper fetal growth and development. All of this sets up both you and your baby for better health and eases healing after your pregnancy. Following the food recommendations outlined later in this chapter will help guide you on how to meet this need.

Studies show you should aim to eat 75 to 100 grams of protein daily. Clinically, I have seen that a more moderate amount of 50 to 80 grams of protein daily can be sufficient if you have an overall healthy diet. If you are a vegetarian, focus should be on balanced complete protein sources while maintaining a warm digestion (for example, combining rice and beans as they contain balanced essential amino acids). More about this can be found in Chapter 4.

▎ Key Supplements

Some supplements are appropriate to incorporate into your diet during pregnancy, but be careful to take the right kinds and right amounts. Many supplements may claim certain amounts of nutrients, but in actuality they may not contain what they claim to. For that reason, it is ideal to obtain supplements from a professional practitioner to ensure quality. Too little or too much of a nutrient can create complications, so it's important to be conscious of the levels of nutrients you are getting both from supplements and diet.

Folic Acid

Consuming B9, also known as folate (from natural food sources) and folic acid (synthetic version) starting early in your pregnancy, or even prior to becoming pregnant, serves a number of important functions in supporting you and your baby's health. It helps make and repair DNA, aids production of red blood cells, and prevents complications such as miscarriage, preeclampsia, and certain birth defects. But how much folate or folic acid you take and where it comes from matters. Because women are advised to take multivitamins containing folic acid before and throughout pregnancy, the supplementation together with natural dietary folates has led to a demographic with high and rising serum levels of unmetabolized folic acid.

Unmetabolized folic acid can also be the result of a genetic metabolic issue leading to hyperhomocysteinemia, or abnormally high levels of amino acids in the blood. This is seen in people with a particular type of gene mutation. When the MTHFR gene malfunctions, folic acid isn't broken down. However, taking the active, converted form of folic acid in the form of L-methylfolate can decrease risks during pregnancy and is easier to metabolize with the gene mutation.

In general, I recommend that my patients take a folic acid supplement in the form of L-methylfolate even if we don't know the status of the gene, as it is more easily metabolized. I also advise them to be conscientious of how much folic acid and/or folate they are consuming through their diet. You can find specific foods and recommended folate levels in the guidelines in the appendix.

DHA

Docosahexaenoic acid (DHA) is a long-chain polyunsaturated fatty acid necessary for normal brain growth and cognitive development. Studies have shown that supplementing with DHA during pregnancy and breastfeeding may have a positive effect on the baby's brain and development.[1]

Raspberry Leaf

Raspberry leaf tea taken throughout a pregnancy helps to strengthen the uterus and regulate hormones to ease hormonal

---

1 Braarud, H. C., Markhus, M. W., Skotheim, S., Stormark, K. M., Frøyland, L., Graff, I. E., & Kjellevold, M. (2018). Maternal DHA status during pregnancy has a positive impact on infant problem solving: A Norwegian prospective observation study. *Nutrients, 10*(5), 529. doi:10.3390/nu10050529.

shifts. It is thought to help with mineral and electrolyte balance that is especially beneficial to the uterine muscles. The tea has been used for hundreds of years to improve labor and delivery outcomes and reduce bleeding postdelivery. Drinking a good quality red raspberry leaf tea throughout pregnancy and especially during the third trimester can provide support and can also be an enjoyable addition to your diet. It is generally recommended to drink about one cup a few times a week during the first two trimesters and up to a quart a day during the last few weeks of your pregnancy to prepare for labor.

Morning Sickness

Many women experience morning sickness (nausea and vomiting) during the first months of their pregnancy. Some theories hold that it is Mother Nature's way of protecting mothers and fetuses from food-borne illness and also shielding the fetus from chemicals that can deform fetal organs at the most critical time in development. A bland diet for the first eight to twelve weeks often helps morning sickness as the immune and digestive systems change during pregnancy, especially the first trimester.

To follow the bland diet, avoid raw or uncooked foods and increase your intake of easily digestible, soft-consistency, cooked foods.

There are different manifestations of morning sickness, and each one has its own remedies and strategies.

Manifestation	Characteristics	Remedies
Deficient	Morning sickness is predominant in the morning, gets better after eating and rest, and you may have slight nausea right after eating, vomit thin fluids, and have an absence of thirst and general aversion to foods.	• Eat small meals more regularly with the focus on proteins, electrolytes, and good fats and oils • Take prenatal vitamins with lunch or dinner instead of in the mornings
Weak Digestion	Combines the deficient manifestation plus leads to dampness in the body with a feeling of fullness, or feeling full quickly, and you may have a sticky taste and excess phlegm, such as runny nose.	See deficient manifestation above plus: • Focus on warming and damp draining foods and drink, such as ginger and ginger tea • Avoid a lot of dairy or raw foods
Excess Stagnation	Morning sickness is predominant in the afternoon, worse after eating, and you feel better with vomiting, feel thirsty with a desire to drink cold fluids, and a bitter or sour taste in the mouth.	• Eat neutral to warming foods while avoiding cooling or hot foods • Cook with ginger • Drink ginger tea
Severe Stagnation	Excess/stagnation manifestation type plus morning sickness with distention and pain, improves with exercise, and you may have sour vomiting, thirst without a desire to drink, irritability, and feeling of fullness in the sternum.	• Drink warm lemon water beginning in the morning throughout the days • Drink raspberry leaf tea, rose hip tea • Eat vinegar-based foods plus excess/stagnation food types

Chapter 1: Prepare

General Strategies for Morning Sickness:

1. Eat bland foods
2. Drink grapefruit peel tea (steep the peel of an organic grapefruit)
3. Have small meals or snacks throughout day
4. Stay hydrated

▰ FOODS THROUGH THE TRIMESTERS

Let's take a look at the nutrients needed throughout the first three trimesters. With each new trimester, you'll incorporate new food groups in addition to the ones added in the previous trimester. Warm digestion principles will also guide food choices to improve health (more information on this in Chapter 4).

▰ First Trimester Foods

Folic Acid: (up to 400ug/day including supplement sources) green leafy veggies, root veggies, whole grains, wheat germ, milk, salmon, nuts

Iron: molasses, whole grains, wheat germ, red meat, poultry, egg yolk, almonds, dried figs, currants, avocados, green leafy veggies

Vitamin A: egg yolk, butter, cheese, yogurt, carrots, spinach, broccoli, apples, mangoes

Vitamin B: egg yolk, molasses, whole grains, wheat germ, rice, legumes, green veggies, bananas, papayas, dried peaches, prunes

Vitamin C: citrus fruits (avoid oranges and orange juice), black currants, melons, pineapples, bananas, raspberries, apples, prunes, tomatoes, potatoes, brussels sprouts, kale, broccoli, parsley, alfalfa, rose hips

Vitamin E: unrefined, cold pressed oils (like olive or flax) whole grains, wheat germ, nuts, green leafy veggies, avocados, molasses, eggs

Zinc: meat, poultry, fish, ginger, sunflower seeds, sesame seeds, pumpkin seeds, sprouted seeds, almonds, soybeans, green leafy veggies, watercress, wheat germ, oat germ, whole grains

Second Trimester Foods

For the most part during the second trimester, you should eat whole, fresh foods and sufficient green veggies (preferably steamed) that will not only provide nutrition but will also reduce swelling.

Generally:

1. Protein intake of 50–80 grams daily

2. Good fats and oils

3. Electrolytes

Foods from the first trimester plus:

Calcium: whole grains, nuts, dairy products, carob, dolomite, green leafy veggies

Chromium: molasses, whole grains, wheat germ, veggies, butter

Essential Fatty Acids: nuts, unrefined oils, nut butters (almond, sesame), green leafy veggies, seeds (sunflower), oily fish (mackerel, tuna)

Magnesium: nuts, kelp, seafood, eggs, milk, whole grains, green veggies, dolomite

Selenium: tuna, herring, butter, wheat germ, brazil nuts, garlic, whole grains

Vitamin D: whole milk, cheese, yogurt, eggs, fish oil, fatty fish

Second and Third Trimester Ailments and Strategies

Reflux

- Drink warm lemon water
- Eat small meals
- Avoid eating close to bedtime
- Avoid inflammatory foods

Constipation

- Drink a glass of unfiltered peach juice (preferably organic) every day

▍Third Trimester Foods

Vitamin K: cauliflower, cabbage, egg yolks, green leafy veggies, soybeans

▍Foods to Avoid or Reduce

As a general rule of thumb, these foods and drinks should be avoided throughout pregnancy:

- Sodas
- Foods containing too much sugar or caffeine
- Saturated fats, such as fried foods
- Foods with additives and preservatives
- Pâté
- Cooked chilled foods, like leftovers
- Undercooked meat
- Uncooked eggs
- Soft or blue-veined or unpasteurized cheese, like Brie or blue cheese, as these carry the risk of infection from salmonella and listeria

Exercise

You should do light exercises throughout your pregnancy to safeguard your pelvic floor and abdominal muscles. Avoid exercises and activities that build too much abdominal pressure in the second and third trimesters (e.g., lifting, crunches, sit-ups, and planks).

Historical Traditional Chinese Medicine Recommendations for Pregnancy

Month 1: eat nourishing and easily digested foods, especially barley

Months 2–3: avoid pungent, hot, and drying foods

Month 4: eat rice, fish, and goose to make the fetus's qi and blood strong

Month 5: eat wheat, beef, and lamb; get extra sleep; spend time in natural sunlight; take baths

Month 6: do light exercises, especially breathing to strengthen fetus's lungs

Month 7: do exercises that flex joints, avoid cold foods, eat rice to nourish fetus's teeth and bones

Month 8: avoid emotional stress and practice quiet breathing to maintain qi and promote lustrous skin in the fetus

Month 9: eat sweet foods, wear loose clothing, avoid dampness, and concentrate qi to lower *dan tian* (a handbreadth below umbilicus) to promote the growth of fetus's joints and mental faculties

Qi is, in simplistic terms, considered an energetic vital force—in our body, in what we eat and drink, in everything around us—that ultimately affects our body's function.

CHAPTER 2: RECOVER

▰ THE FOURTH TRIMESTER

The first three trimesters are all about optimizing your health to support your baby, but the fourth trimester is about optimizing your health so you can heal. Proper healing supports breastfeeding (if you are doing this) and enhances your ability to care for your newborn. It also has a positive downstream effect for the health and social outcomes of the whole family across their lifetimes.

Sadly, postpartum care in the United States is notoriously lacking. We have an uphill battle with the current structures in health care, jobs, and politics along with the prevailing cultural norms. I believe we are ready to turn that tide and support women and their families in this particularly vulnerable and critical time.

> "The United States is the only developed nation in the world lacking public policies that support women with some kind of paid compensation after giving birth, such as maternity leave or financial assistance if they don't have a job."
>
> —*The First Forty Days: The Essential Art of Nourishing the New Mother*

■ A MATTER OF LIFE OR DEATH

After childbirth, in the United States, it is standard for a postpartum woman to have her first checkup six weeks after the baby is born. As we have discussed already, this is a particularly vulnerable time for the woman and also a very important time for healing. "An estimated 700 women die in the U.S. every year from causes related to pregnancy and childbirth. That's more than in any other country in the developed world. Another 65,000 *nearly* die. And women of color are particularly vulnerable, according to the Centers for Disease Control and Prevention."[2] While the data do not clearly point to direct causes of pregnancy-related deaths, we know that the postpartum period plays an important role as the definition of this category of health outcomes includes the entire first year of pregnancy.

To address the unacceptably high maternal mortality rate, the American College of Obstetricians and Gynecologists recently released guidelines suggesting that a new mom's first doctor visit should come within three weeks of delivery. This is a step in the right direction, but in my opinion still falls vastly short of what is needed to address this gap in health care for women.

No matter what your circumstances are, you deserve to have a healthy and well-supported pregnancy *and* postpartum. The hope of this book is to present a commonsense approach to healing along with the necessary information to best understand how your body functions, what red flags to look for, and the simple steps you can take to support your own healing.

---

2 Cheng, C. Y., Fowles, E. R., & Walker, L. O. (2006). Continuing education module: postpartum maternal health care in the United States: A critical review. *The Journal of Perinatal Education, 15*(3), 34–42.

▍ THE FIRST 10 DAYS[3]

Nobody *really* tells you what changes to expect in your body after giving birth beyond basic information. I know that was the case when I had my first baby, even though health care providers surrounded me—including a team of three midwives—and I was studying East Asian medicine and had already completed the obstetrics rotation as part of my training. If I had known then what I know now, that knowledge would have helped me sort through whether my feelings were normal or whether it was something I should worry about. I think it is almost impossible to truly prepare for the physical effects you will experience with your first baby when you literally feel like you've been hit by a Mack truck. Experiencing postpartum for the first time can also make you feel guilty that it is not all "easy." After all, women have been doing this as long as there have been humans, right?! Even if you can never be fully prepared for what postpartum will feel like, having a better understanding of your body and the healing process will empower you to feel secure in your experience and your decisions.

"Nobody told me I would still look pregnant after giving birth."

Uterus. After giving birth, the uterus starts to return to its pre-pregnancy size through the process of involution (shrinking back to size). After birth, the uterus is about the height of the belly button, and about one week later it's the height of the pubic bone. The lining of the uterus, called the lochia, begins to shed after delivery, which will result in bleeding and cramping. You can help this process by gently massaging your uterus a few times a day until you feel it contract and harden. You can find the top of your uterus by gently pressing down from your umbilicus toward your pubic bone until you feel a hardening—that is the uterus. Gently massage for a few minutes until you feel the

---

3 Adapted from *Acupuncture in Pregnancy and Childbirth* by Zita West

defined hardening, which is a sign it is contracting. If bleeding or cramping becomes consistent, this is a sign that you may be doing too much too soon. Doing too much can include standing, lifting, and walking more than you should, which can also put too much burden on the healing uterus. If this is happening, get off your feet and rest. If you develop a fever, you should call your doctor right away as this might indicate an infection or retention of lochia.

In my practice, I recommend Chinese herb formulas to my patients to help with returning the uterus to normal and clearing the lochia. This is a very specific treatment, so it is best to seek a qualified acupuncture and Chinese herbalist practitioner.

"Nobody told me how sore my nipples would be with breastfeeding."

Breasts. After birth, the secretion of the hormone (prolactin) initiates the production of milk (lactation). For the first few days, the breast milk is made up of mostly colostrum, which is considered the ultimate superfood for your new baby. After about two to five days, your milk will become a mixture of mature milk and colostrum. Your breasts can become temporarily engorged, and it is helpful to consult with a lactation specialist if you're having breastfeeding problems. If your nipples become sore or cracked, you can use a balm to help soothe and heal the discomfort. Prevention goes a long way. It's a good idea to source a high-quality nipple cream you can use with breastfeeding and apply it right away before your nipples become dry or cracked.

Breast Surgery. If you've had any kind of breast surgery, you should talk to your doctor or lactation specialist as this can result in complications with breastfeeding. Early on in my practice, I worked with a patient who had had breast reductions. When she had her baby, she still produced some milk but not enough to maintain a healthy weight gain for the baby. This was complicated by the fact that her baby preferred breastfeeding and refused a bottle. If we had anticipated that the breast reduction surgery would be related to complications with milk production, we could have adjusted her plan to help the baby acclimate to a bottle early on.

Mastitis. One of the more common challenges that moms will experience is mastitis, which is inflammation of the breast tissue that can lead to an infection. To prevent this, allow yourself time to rest and heal postpartum. Stress and overdoing it can contribute to making you more vulnerable to mastitis. If you experience a redness or pain in the breast tissue, consult your doctor right away.

Colostrum. Typically, you produce about one to four teaspoons of colostrum each day. For moms who can't breastfeed or situations where the newborn is unable to get colostrum through breast milk, there are colostrum supplementation options to add to baby formula. Check with your pediatrician or lactation specialist for the best supplement options. Some of the important health benefits for your baby include:

- Helps your baby build a strong immune system by transmitting antibodies and white blood cells.

- Creates a tough coating on your baby's stomach and intestines to keep germs from causing illness.

- Acts as a laxative to help your baby pass meconium (the dark first poop).

- Helps prevent jaundice (yellowing of the skin) and gets rid of harmful waste products.

- Gives your baby's brain, eyes, and heart the right blend of nutrients to grow.

- Contains high levels of protein, salts, fats, and vitamins for complete nutrition.

- Provides nutrients that your baby's stomach can easily digest.

- Helps to prevent low blood sugar in newborns.

There are so many scenarios with breastfeeding. For some moms, the process will be easy and for others it will be more challenging for a variety of reasons. The most important thing is to never feel guilty about choosing what is best for you and your baby given all the factors that are unique to you.

"Nobody told me how sore I would be after a vaginal birth."

Perineum. If you've had a vaginal delivery, the perineum (the area between the vagina and anus) can be very sore and take some time to heal, especially if you had a tear that required stitches. You might also experience soreness or discomfort in the lower part of the anus (hemorrhoids), since pushing can cause the veins to swell and become painful and itchy.

Bladder. You can expect a marked increase in urination after delivery as your body begins to return to pre-pregnant fluid levels and return to normal blood volume. If this isn't occurring and you feel that your urinary tract has been strained, it is good to check with your doctor sooner rather than later.

Bowels. Your bowel movements can be affected whether you've had a C-section or vaginal birth. If you don't return to normal (i.e., having at least one bowel movement per day) within a couple days after giving birth, you should start taking steps to try to get back on a daily bowel movement schedule. You'll find remedies in Chapter 4 for softening stools and promoting healthy bowels by following the warm digestion principles postpartum.

Muscles. It takes up to three months (the entirety of the fourth trimester) for the pelvic joints, ligaments, and muscles that have softened during pregnancy to return to normal. This is why resting and not overexerting yourself or doing heavy lifting is so important during this healing time.

"Nobody told me about the night sweats."

Hormones. The postpartum hormone drop is the single largest sudden hormone change in the shortest amount of time that a woman will ever experience. During pregnancy, estrogen and progesterone increase to levels equivalent to taking a hundred birth control pills a day. Around three days postpartum, your hormones essentially return to baseline levels. This dramatic shift in estrogen and progesterone can cause huge emotional and physiological changes and can be marked with night sweats, fatigue, digestive changes, anxiety, and the general feeling of riding an emotional rollercoaster, just to name a few. Resting and eating well can help you recover and smooth out this time of intense transition.

"Nobody told me I would fantasize about sleep."

Sleep and Healing. When I had my son, I was not prepared for what it would be like to have regular and consistent loss of sleep. People offer casual comments about the lack of sleep as a new parent, but no one really tells you what that sleeplessness does to you. Let's be honest: Sleep deprivation is a form of torture. I used to fantasize about sleep after I had my son, who would not sleep more than three hours at a time for the first year. I was young, and it didn't even cross my mind to seek help for sleep training or to get support for this very important issue. Worse, once my son started sleeping better, I would still wake up every three hours because my body was stuck in that pattern. Persistent loss of sleep can make you more vulnerable to postpartum depression. Another new mom shared her experience with me:

> When I had my first baby, I used to get very blue around 8 PM (summer) when the sun started to come down because everyone else in the household was getting ready to rest, and I knew I was facing a sleepless night (my baby slept during the day and not a blink at night). It took me 10 months to gather the strength to let her cry it out. She cried for five minutes and went to sleep through the night ever since!

Please be proactive and take steps to protect your sleep. Adequate rest is essential to postpartum healing, and finding the right tools may require extra support.

General Remedies and Strategies

- Massage the uterus every day to help it return to normal.
- Consult with a lactation consultant for extra guidance.
- Use balm on sore or cracked nipples.
- Wash with a perineal bottle, soak in sitz baths, and apply witch hazel pads to help heal the perineum.
- Rest and avoid heavy lifting to allow muscles time to return to normal.
- Try warm digestion principles for irregular bowel movements.

▪ WHEN TO SEEK MEDICAL ATTENTION

Adapted from *The Essential Guide to Acupuncture in Pregnancy and Childbirth* by Debra Betts

If you notice any of these changes in your body, you should call your health care provider. These may be signs of more serious complications that need extra support and treatment.

1. Heavy bleeding after the first 12 hours.

2. Persistent red, heavy bleeding after the first four days.

3. Foul-smelling discharge.

4. Discharge containing large blood clots.

5. Discharge entirely absent the first two weeks.

6. Persistent abdominal pain.

7. Raised temperature after the first 24 hours.

8. Pain, warmth, or tenderness in the calf muscle.

9. Sudden, sharp chest pain with or without difficulty breathing.

10. Persistent oozing at a C-section scar.

11. Pain, swelling, redness, and feeling of heat in the breast accompanied by general chills, fever, or flu-like symptoms.

12. Severe or prolonged depression.

CHAPTER 3: HEAL

▎KICK GUILT TO THE CURB

Nobody expects someone who has just undergone surgery to return immediately to full capacity. Yet, for some reason, the expectation for new moms is that they will have a baby, jump out of bed, and get back to normal, all while caring for a newborn baby on very little sleep. Society certainly plays a role in this, and perhaps we place this expectation on ourselves, too.

I get it. I had my son during acupuncture and Chinese Medicine school and had to take exams three weeks after he was born. That's just the way it was. I remember crying my eyes out in the shower at 4:30 in the morning before a pharmacology exam, because I was just so exhausted. Luckily, since I was in school, I had a few tools in my toolkit that helped me recover during this time: Chinese herb formulas, acupuncture, and warming, nourishing foods. Even with the right tools, it's still hard to give ourselves permission to rest and to not buy into the false expectation that we should bounce back immediately. I jumped back into school and worked too quickly out of fear of falling behind, and I know now that it was not the best approach. I was young and headstrong, and, if I had to do it over again, I would take my postpartum recovery more seriously. Be gentle with yourself, accept help, and let yourself heal.

▎HEALING BASICS

Proper healing is essential for getting back to life, including exercise and work. If you give yourself a chance to heal, you have better odds of successfully "re-entering" life in whatever capacity it demands. Following these guiding principles as much as you are able to will help you heal:

- Eat warming and nourishing foods (we'll go into more detail about this in Chapter 4).

- Especially during the first month, take good care of your abdomen by resting as much as possible, using an abdominal wrap, not lifting anything heavier than the newborn baby, and staying warm (not getting chilled).

- If you had a vaginal birth, take care of the perineum with perineal bottle washes after going to the bathroom and regular sitz baths.

- If you had a C-section, follow your doctor's advice and be very careful about lifting and doing too much too soon.

- If you are feeling better (after four weeks for vaginal births and six weeks for C-sections), you can begin to incorporate light exercise like walking and postnatal yoga or Pilates to restore your core strength.

- Look into additional specialists—like acupuncturists/Chinese Medicine practitioners, pelvic floor and lactation specialists, postpartum doulas—to further support your recovery.

▰ POSTPARTUM RESTING

You need rest to heal, especially during the first month after giving birth. This means staying horizontal for most of the day to give your abdomen and pelvic floor a chance to heal. Try to avoid picking anything up heavier than your newborn. Only consider light exercise such as gentle walking when you've reached <u>six weeks</u> postpartum. You'll need to wait longer than six weeks if you've had a C-section or any other complications. In the second to third months postpartum, you can resume your core exercises.

Avoid any impact exercises where you are "bouncing your pelvic floor," like running or jumping, until you are fully healed, which typically happens in the fourth month. Healing might take longer if you had a C-section, experienced significant tears that required stitches, or had other complications. While this may feel impossible—especially if you have more than one child, a job, or other unavoidable responsibilities—I cannot stress enough how important proper rest is for your short- and long-term health.

ABDOMINAL WRAPPING

Abdominal wrapping is worn during the day until the abdomen has returned to size and is used in many cultures postpartum beginning about five days after giving birth. The practice helps support healing and protects the vulnerable abdomen and pelvic floor during this recovery period. Women around the world have been belly wrapping their bodies after childbirth for years. Wrapping the belly and waist tightly after delivery can help speed recovery. There are many good products available as awareness grows. I recommend an adjustable compression-style belly wrap that is designed to reduce swelling and help support your core abdominal muscles while you recover from childbirth.

Abdominal wrapping can also help the separation of abdominal muscles heal. It is common for the two muscles that run down the middle of your stomach to separate during pregnancy. This is called diastasis recti. The separation should return to normal about eight weeks postpartum. A way to check the amount of separation is to lie on your back with legs bent, feet flat on the floor. Raise your shoulders off the floor slightly and look at your abdomen. Palpate the edges of your muscles in the abdomen with your fingers and see if you can fit fingers into the gap between the muscles. If this hasn't closed by eight weeks postpartum, it is a good idea to consult with a specialist, explained later in this chapter for pelvic floor and abdominal healing.[4]

---

[4] United Kingdom National Health Service. (2019, October 22). Your post-pregnancy body. Retrieved from https://www.nhs.uk/conditions/pregnancy-and-baby/your-body-after-childbirth/.

Patient Story: Diastasis Recti

JP came to me in her late 30s during assisted fertility treatment when she was attempting to get pregnant with her second child. Through acupuncture and assisted fertility, she became pregnant with twins. She continued to see me regularly throughout her pregnancy for acupuncture and guidance with Chinese herb formulas and nutrition. She carried her twin boys to full term and had a C-section at 39 weeks. Following the birth, she experienced severe diastasis recti where the muscles were so separated that, no matter how much treatment we did afterwards, the abdominal muscles would not fully heal back together. She continued with herbs and acupuncture to support her healing until she felt strong enough to have corrective surgery four years later (she also had an underlying autoimmune disease, which complicated this decision). She continued acupuncture during postoperative healing and made a full recovery. I am including this story because I think it's important to understand the support one can experience with acupuncture and the whole system of Chinese Medicine whilst, at the same time, seek the care one needs with surgery or other practices modern Western medicine has to offer. In this case, no amount of restoring the core or acupuncture was going to heal the separation of the muscles, but it did allow her to reach a point where she could handle the surgery and heal successfully.

■ VAGINAL BIRTHS

After a vaginal birth, you will have soreness and swelling. If you've had an episiotomy or stitches from a tear, it will take longer to heal. Some strategies make the healing process easier. Your perineum, the area between your vagina and anus, will have been stretched and bruised and will need special care. It's also common to have hemorrhoids, or painful swelling in the anus or rectum. Using a perineal spray bottle to clean yourself with every bathroom visit until you're healed is really helpful and reduces pain. Sitz baths also are very soothing and help cleanse and heal the tissue. A sitz bath is a shallow bath for your perineum. You can obtain a shallow bowl that fits in your toilet seat or you can fill your bathtub with shallow water. It is important to keep either the bath or shallow bowl clean between soaks. If you are experiencing a lot of pain, you can use witch hazel pads both on the perineum and rectum. Sitting on a donut-shaped pillow the first couple weeks will keep any unnecessary pressure off your swollen tissue. If you experience pain for longer than the average time for vaginal healing after birth (six weeks), it's very important to consult your doctor and not live with the pain. Extensive tearing and stitches may take up to 12 weeks to heal. However, if you still experience pain when you should be healed, your tissue may be unevenly healing and creating bunching. Regardless, it is important to fully heal before resuming sex or vigorous exercise. According to Chinese Medicine, you would want your vaginal tissue to be fully healed before using tampons and exposure to cold water (such as swimming) as well.

Patient Story: Vaginal Birth Recovery

LB came to my clinic about a year after the birth of her first daughter. She was suffering from chronic sacroiliac and sacral pain, which we addressed. A year later, she wanted to have a second child. She became pregnant, and I continued to provide care throughout her pregnancy to manage, among other things, stabilizing her low back and pelvis during the pregnancy. She had an uncomplicated vaginal birth, and I continued to see her postpartum. She noted how much better her second pregnancy and postpartum healing went compared to her first pregnancy. She experienced less pain and overwhelm, even with the added challenge of now having a toddler and a newborn baby.

▪ CESAREAN SECTION (C-SECTION) BIRTHS

Cesarean section (C-section) births come with the added complication of major surgery. While it is critical to follow your surgeon's directions, you can find additional healing and pain relief with Chinese herb formulas, acupuncture, and abdominal wrapping. The most important thing to do is rest. You should not lift anything heavier than your newborn during the first few weeks; when you feed your baby, using a pillow under your arm can provide extra support. Acupuncture can be very helpful with healing the incision, reducing swelling, pain, and numbness, and minimizing the appearance of the incision scar.

Patient Story: C-section

NJ came to see me for help with fertility for her third child, and I continued to work with her throughout the pregnancy. She had a C-section without complications at 40 weeks. I continued to see her postpartum and regularly treated and addressed her surgical incision. This was her third C-section, and her previous surgeries had left her in a lot of pain with numbness around the incision. One area of the C-section took longer to heal, but seeing her weekly enabled a full healthy recovery with less pain and numbness. It was a good reminder to me about the importance of continued treatment for C-section scar treatments for healing to prevent the progression of potentially serious complications.

■ NIPPLE CARE

There are some very good nipple balms on the market to soothe and soften nursing nipples. I would recommend having this on hand before you give birth and using it preventively, if you know you will try breastfeeding. Choose one that you don't have to wash off before breastfeeding and is safe for the baby.

■ STRETCH MARKS

Prevention goes a long way in reducing the appearance of stretch marks. Using a pregnancy belly cream product that contains shea butter on your abdomen and anywhere else you are prone to stretch marks—such as hips, thighs, upper arms, and breasts—will help to increase hydration and enhance elasticity to allow the skin to stretch without tearing the dermis (which is what causes stretch marks). This is especially important in your third trimester when the most growth happens. Adequate levels of good fats, oils, and proteins to nourish your skin during pregnancy are helpful, such as olive oil, butter, avocados, nuts, whole eggs, and natural meats, to name a few.

A technique that I like for postpartum healing of stretch marks, abdomen muscles, balancing hormones, and helping the body back to health in general is an Ayurvedic warm oil called Abhyanga.[5] Warm oil, which is sometimes medicated with herbs, is gently massaged over the entire body in a certain pattern before bathing. Abhyanga can also calm the nervous system and make a profound difference for a sleep-deprived postpartum mom.

> **Patient Story: Stretch Marks**
>
> TL gave birth vaginally to an eight-pound, five-ounce baby girl. I had seen her throughout her pregnancy as well as postpartum. During her pregnancy, she had developed significant stretch marks across the lower part of her abdomen that were causing her distress. Along with other postpartum care, we used acupuncture to treat her stretch marks for the first few months postpartum. As she continued to heal, the stretch marks faded and improved so much that they are no longer visible. I find it incredibly rewarding to help new moms heal and recover with all the challenges that pregnancy brings.

---

5 Welch, Claudia. (2011). *Balance your hormones, balance your life: achieving optimal health and wellness through Ayurveda, Chinese medicine, and western science.* Boston: Da Capo Lifelong Books.

■ PELVIC FLOOR RECOVERY

Pelvic floor muscles play an essential role in your health by supporting the uterus, bladder, and bowels, and the physical changes throughout pregnancy certainly take a toll on them. Studies have found that delivery results in partial denervation (loss of nerve supply) of the pelvic floor in most women.[6] Complications or inadequate healing can lead to incontinence or leaking. It can also result in prolapse, which occurs when the pelvic organs lack sufficient support and begin to fall into or out of the vagina. Even if you don't suffer from incontinence or prolapse after delivery, your core and pelvic floor need to recover, realign, and regain strength after having a baby. It is really important to start this process before resuming physical activities and sports that put any impact on the pelvic floor, such as running or jumping. Further, adequate healing can help prevent injury, pain, and complications later in life

To retrain the pelvic floor muscles, you can do Kegel exercises at home. The goal is to strengthen the pelvic floor by contracting and relaxing the muscles in your vagina. It can be challenging to identify the right muscles and to know whether you are working them in the right way. One helpful trick is to imagine that there is a straw in your vagina and you are trying to suck liquid up through the straw. If you feel tightening in that area, then you have successfully found your pelvic floor muscles. You'll probably notice that they fatigue easily at first. Keep up with the exercises throughout the day to improve their strength. You can also seek out specialists such as pelvic floor physical therapists, acupuncture practitioners, and Pilates trainers to help address the pelvic floor healing. As your abdomen heals, it will also help stabilize the pelvic floor.

---

6 Allen, R., Hosker G. L., Smith, A. R. B. & Warrell, D. W. (1990). Pelvic floor damage and childbirth: A neurophysiological study. *BJOG: An International Journal of Obstetrics & Gynaecology*, 97, 770–779.

EXERCISE AND LOSING THE "BABY WEIGHT"

In the first six months postpartum, low impact cardio is preferred over running, jumping, and heavy weights. Your body has lingering elevated levels of relaxin, which keep your muscles more pliable and susceptible to injury. It's okay to move and get your heart rate up to burn calories, but be cautious of your joints.[7]

It is *very* important not to do any strenuous exercise that gets your heart rate up and puts impact on your pelvic floor until after month three postpartum. This is considered the end of the fourth trimester, which is all about healing the mother. If you are feeling good and strong after the fourth trimester, you can start sensibly getting back to your normal exercise routine. If you have given yourself enough time to heal, you will be amazed how easy it is to get back to normal life and still feel good. Not only that, but you will find that, as your body properly heals, it naturally begins to shed the "baby weight." Once you pass the threshold and have the ability to fully get back to regular exercise, you will be able to reach your weight goals with reduced risk of injuries or setbacks.

SPECIALISTS

Acupuncture and Chinese Medicine Practitioner

Acupuncture and Chinese Medicine can be very effective in supporting proper healing postpartum and has been used for thousands of years to treat women during this crucial time. More and more Western women are discovering for themselves the benefits it offers for their health. As a practitioner, my years in practice have shown me that it can be a real game changer when it comes to certain unresolved issues. Modern telehealth opens

---

[7] Ardnt, Laura. (2020). Healthy pelvic floor muscles start during pregnancy. Retrieved from https://bloomlife.com/preg-u/healthy-pelvic-floor-muscles-start-pregnancy/.

up so many doors for patients, who can now be seen remotely if they do not have childcare or cannot come into the clinic for any reason. I cannot stress enough that if you have any unresolved issues, getting treatment can be helpful for many months or even **years** after giving birth. I not only regularly treat women postpartum but also can trace improper healing postpartum up to years and decades after childbirth. Common issues I see in my practice include (but are not limited to): chronic pain (particularly in the pelvis, low back, or sciatic nerve), anxiety, insomnia, difficult transitions to menopause, incontinence and urinary issues, endocrine issues, hormonal issues, abdominal and core strength issues, prolapse, and even jaw pain and migraines.

In my own clinic, I routinely give my patients Chinese herb formulas to help the uterus clear and contract to a normal position as well as formulas designed to smooth out the hormonal transition, support breastfeeding, and safeguard overall health. If postpartum moms have the luxury of making the time to come into my clinic, acupuncture treatment is very helpful for healing after the "resting month." Patients who have come in for treatment during their pregnancy, taken herbs for postpartum, followed the warm digestion principle, and come in even just once or twice postpartum have remarked that they have had a better time recovering than prior pregnancies without support.

I was pregnant with my son in my last year of acupuncture and Chinese Medicine school. Back then, everyone was reticent about treating with acupuncture during pregnancy (fortunately, that is not the case anymore). Once I graduated, I was determined to learn what hadn't translated yet to our American education. Thanks to the acupuncture/midwife combined training and authors and educators such as Zita West and Debra Betts, I realized there is a long tradition for pregnancy and postpartum support. Consequently, I dedicated myself to include extensive maternal health in my practice and have truly enjoyed following patients through pregnancy and postpartum and witnessing the positive effects daily. Ideally, I see patients weekly through the first trimester and then on a monthly basis until they reach 30 weeks if there are no complications in their pregnancy. After 30 weeks, I see them more frequently again to help them through the last trimester and prep them for labor, delivery, and postpartum.

If you're looking for a practitioner, it is always a good idea to ask them if they specialize in pregnancy and postpartum support. Ask specifically about "mother warming," a technique that uses moxa (Chinese herb with the genus *Artemisia*) to energize and facilitate healing. Acupuncture and Chinese Medicine is a growing field in the United States and around the world. It is well equipped to support women at this stage and works synergistically with Western medicine. I find that using the two approaches together achieves the best of both worlds.

How to Find an Acupuncturist

- Search the National Certification Commission for Acupuncture and Oriental Medicine directory at www.nccaom.org
- Internet search "acupuncture" and "women's health" in your area.
- Ask your healthcare providers, friends and/or family for for recommendations.

▰ Pelvic Floor Specialist

Pelvic floor specialists can help support your recovery process by guiding you through exercises and incorporating other techniques to support healing. The best time to see a specialist is eight weeks after giving birth. While the importance of addressing the pelvic floor is becoming more widely known, it is rarely suggested or recommended in the United States. unless there is a significant issue. Some countries, like France, provide government-sponsored physical therapy to support pelvic floor muscle recovery as a standard part of postnatal care. I certainly would like it to be standard care for postpartum women and believe it would go a long way to preventing longstanding issues. In the United States, there are physical therapists who specialize in pelvic floor recovery and are a great resource for specialized care.

> **Patient Story: Pelvic Floor**
>
> WJ, a 52-year-old woman, came in for chronic sciatic and low back pain that she had been struggling with for many years. We eventually determined that this pain started after she gave birth to her twins, who were now grown. Between treatment from a pelvic floor specialist and acupuncture, the chronic pain improved. As long as she adhered to specific core-restoring exercises, her pain stayed away.

▪ Postpartum Doula

A postpartum doula provides evidenced-based information on topics such as infant feeding, emotional and physical recovery from birth, mother-baby bonding, infant soothing, and basic newborn care. Research shows that moms, dads, and babies have an easier time with this transition if a good support team is in place. The big benefit here is having a knowledgeable professional right in your home supporting you. Simply priceless.

Patient Story: Postpartum Doula

GM came to me for fertility, and I continued to see her throughout the pregnancy. She had a very complicated pregnancy due to an underlying autoimmune disease, which led to placental lakes and placenta previa. We successfully treated her to 37 weeks. In assessing next steps, we discussed the possibility of a postpartum doula as the best use of her resources for postpartum healing. This is the route she took, and both she and baby had no further complications and have been thriving.

Lactation Specialist

Lactation consultants are nursing professionals who help new moms in their efforts to breastfeed and also provide prenatal education and preparation for expecting couples. Simply put: A lactation specialist can aid you in all your breastfeeding needs.

One patient shared her story with me:

> If I hadn't consulted with a lactation specialist, I wouldn't have been able to breastfeed my first baby. My milk did not come down until day five and the nurses were pushing hard for formula right away even though latching was going well. My baby was hungry and losing weight rapidly. I called the lactation consultant that had trained me from the hospital bed and asked for her advice. We settled on giving her a small amount of formula between breast-feedings until I started producing enough milk. It was stressful to navigate those days, and she really helped me figure things out.

▮ Postpartum Depression Specialists

Postpartum depression (PPD) is a serious issue during the postpartum period. New moms may not be aware of the symptoms they are experiencing, so ask a family member or support person to keep tabs on you to help you identify if you might be in need of professional support from a specialist, including a therapist. Ongoing exhaustion, loss of sleep, and stressful living conditions can deplete anyone and increase the risk for depression. Women who have experienced depression before pregnancy are 20 percent more likely to experience PPD, and as many as 50 to 75 percent of postpartum women will experience the "baby blues." In Traditional Chinese Medicine, healing properly postpartum is one of your strongest preventive measures you can take to avoid PPD.

> **Know the Signs of PPD** [8]
>
> - Persistent sad, anxious, or "empty" mood
> - Irritability
> - Feelings of guilt, worthlessness, hopelessness, or helplessness
> - Loss of interest or pleasure in hobbies and activities
> - Fatigue or abnormal decrease in energy
> - Feeling restless or having trouble sitting still
> - Difficulty concentrating, remembering, or making decisions
> - Difficulty sleeping (even when the baby is sleeping), waking early in the morning, or oversleeping

---

8 National Institute of Mental Health. (2020). Perinatal depression. Retrieved from https://www.nimh.nih.gov/health/publications/perinatal-depression/index.shtml.

- Abnormal appetite, weight changes, or both
- Aches or pains, headaches, cramps, or digestive problems that do not have a clear physical cause or do not ease even with treatment
- Trouble bonding or forming an emotional attachment with the new baby
- Persistent doubts about the ability to care for the new baby
- Thoughts about death, suicide, or harming oneself or the baby

▪ New Fathers Can Get Postpartum Depression, Too

Studies have shown that new fathers can experience postpartum depression as well, and at least 25 percent of men may experience PPD in the first two months of a newborn's life.

Anecdotally, I have heard from many patients about their experiences with partners being temporarily or permanently affected by witnessing the traumatic delivery and developing generalized panic and anxiety. One patient shared that her husband literally went to sleep for two weeks after the birth of their first child and felt abandoned by her attention to the baby. Perhaps by acknowledging that the postpartum period is a significant transition for new fathers, we can be prepared to help men get support when needed.

▪ Baby Sleep Consultants

Sleep is such a critical component for your, your baby's, and your family's health. There are many options for specialist support, including therapists, coaches, and night nannies. Check with your pediatrician for more information. You will do yourself and your baby a favor if you learn how to sleep better from the beginning.

■ BENEFITS OF SUPPORT

One of the biggest benefits of continued support during and after pregnancy, my patients often say, is that it calms their anxiety and worry. Getting support during postpartum helps you feel less overwhelmed and more heard. It also helps you navigate any complications or issues with professional help sooner rather than later.

CHAPTER 4: NOURISH

It's hard to underscore just how important it is to focus on your nutrition during the postpartum period, especially during the fourth trimester. At the same time, this is also one of the most challenging times to do so. If you prepare prior to giving birth, it will go a long way to support you the first month. The more you can organize, the easier this can be.

In my practice, I teach new moms the principles behind eating warm and nourishing foods. This helps their bodies to heal and supports breastfeeding. It also helps newborns develop healthy digestion and reduces the possibility of colic and other digestive upsets.

■ WHAT IS WARM DIGESTION?

The concept of keeping a warm digestion is deeply rooted in East Asian medicine. Think of your digestive system as a soup pot that needs to reach a certain temperature to begin to "cook" (or properly digest) the food. All foods, herbs, and spices are categorized and have a temperature ranging from cold to hot. Cooking and certain ways of preparing food, such as adding spices, can help change the temperature qualities of some foods. For example, iced water is cold, but you can warm water to a neutral room temperature or you can boil it to make it hot. The more "cool" foods and drinks you have, the harder your digestive system must work in order to "heat" the food to properly digest. East Asian medicine has shown that keeping a warm digestion during the postpartum period is very important for both the health of the mother and baby.

■ WHY DON'T YOU WANT COOL DIGESTION?

If your digestion is cool or cold, your ability to properly digest food is weakened. You may physically feel the effects of a cool digestion as: slow healing after childbirth, slow to lose the pregnancy weight, irregular digestion, and fatigue. If you are breastfeeding, this may also affect the digestion of your newborn, manifesting as: gas, bloating, colic, or reflux (frequent spitting up).

HOW DO YOU KEEP YOUR DIGESTION WARM?

East Asian medicine is about seeking balance in all areas of life, including food and digestion. Having a nice mix of temperatures, flavors, and foods greatly enhances health.

8 Ways You Can Have Warm Digestion on a Daily Basis During the Fourth Trimester

1. Start your day with a warm, cooked breakfast. Include warming proteins with your breakfast.

2. Drink only warm or room temperature beverages.

3. Eat lots of soups and stews, such as bone broth soup, miso soup, chicken soup, and beef stew.

4. Avoid eating leftovers right out of the refrigerator without warming.

5. Avoid all raw vegetables until four months after giving birth.

6. When eating dairy, choose drier and harder cheeses (less damp and cooling) and plain or neutral flavors of yogurt. Adding cinnamon to yogurt will warm it up.

7. Avoid all fruits until two months after giving birth and then only more warming and in-season or cooked fruits.

8. Avoid most foods on the inflammatory list until month four after giving birth.

▌General Guidelines

- Fruits are cooler than vegetables.

- Vegetables are cooler than grains and legumes.

- Grains, legumes, and nuts are neutral.

- Animal meats are warm.

Within each category though, there is a range of temperatures. Grains, legumes, and nuts are neutral, soy is cooler than rice, and rice is cooler than oats. During the postpartum period, especially the fourth trimester, avoid all cold or cool foods and only eat neutral to warm foods. Let's go through examples of the temperatures of foods within each category.

Fruits

- **Cold:** banana, blueberry, cantaloupe, cranberry, grapefruit, mango, persimmon, rhubarb, tomato, watermelon, mulberry, plum, kiwi

- **Cool:** apple, avocado, black currant, prune, tangerine, pear, oranges, coconut

- **Neutral:** apricot, loquat, papaya, pomegranate, tangerine, peach, lemon

- **Warm:** blackberry, cherry, date, grape, lychee, longan, quince, raspberry, strawberry, kumquat, fig

- **Hot:** pineapple

Vegetables

During postpartum, you can eat from the entire list but you must cook the foods first. However, avoid nightshade vegetables, such bell peppers, tomatoes, and eggplant, as they may affect your breast milk and can upset your baby's digestion.

- **Cold:** asparagus, Chinese cabbage, seaweed, snow pea, water chestnut, dandelion leaf, white mushroom

- **Cool:** artichoke, bok choy, broccoli, cauliflower, celery, corn, cucumber, daikon radish, eggplant, mushroom, spinach, swiss chard, turnip, zucchini, alfalfa sprouts, bamboo shoots, carrot, endive, potato, romaine lettuce, tomato

- **Neutral:** beet, carrot, cabbage, lettuce, shitake mushroom, olive, peas, pumpkin, yam

- **Warm:** bell pepper, chive, green bean, kale, leek, mustard green, parsley, parsnip, squash, sweet potato, watercress, scallions, onion, fennel, oyster mushroom

- **Hot:** garlic, green onion

Grains, Legumes, and Nuts

- **Cold:** wheat germ

- **Cool:** amaranth, barley, buckwheat, millet, wheat, wild rice, lima bean, mung bean, soybean

- **Neutral:** brown rice, corn, flax, white rice, almond, chickpea, hazelnut, peanut, pistachio, pumpkin, sunflower seed

- **Warm:** oat, quinoa, safflower, spelt, black bean, chestnut, pine nut, sesame seed, walnut

Animal Products

- **Cold:** clam, crab, octopus

- **Cool:** eggs, pork, duck

- **Neutral:** abalone, rabbit, cheese, duck, goose, herring, mackerel, cow milk, oyster, salmon, sardine, shark, tuna, chicken

- **Warm:** beef, liver, anchovy, butter, chicken, eel, ham, lobster, mussel, shrimp, turkey, venison, fresh-water fish, sheep, goat, sheep milk

- **Hot:** lamb, trout

■ **Spices and Oils**

- **Cold:** salt, white pepper

- **Cool:** marjoram, mint, peppermint, tamarind, cilantro leaf, sesame oil

- **Neutral:** coriander, licorice, saffron, olive oil, peanut oil

- **Warm:** anise, basil, bay leaf, carob, caraway, clove, cumin, dill seed, fennel, fenugreek, fresh ginger, nutmeg, oregano, rosemary, sage, spearmint, thyme, jasmine, coriander

- **Hot:** black pepper, cayenne pepper, chili pepper, cinnamon, dry ginger, horseradish, wasabi, mustard, garlic

By now, you may be beginning to have a better idea about warm and cold foods. This is by no means an exhaustive list. You can take these lists and experiment and even add your own foods as well. At the end of the day, you are the best judge of your body. For more in-depth information, consider my book, *The Key to a Healthy Digestion: How to Eat Warm and Cold Foods to Improve Your Health*.

■ **Other Nutrient Concerns:**

1. *Protein.* You should consume at least 50 grams of warming proteins daily.

2. *Electrolytes.* Aim to have at least 8 to 12 ounces of balanced electrolytes daily.

3. *Oils.* Include DHA in your supplements as well as one teaspoon of good olive oil daily.

4. *Salt.* Season food with sea salt or high-quality mined salt.

5. *Beverages.* Limit your beverages to warm teas and drinks, and avoid cold or iced drinks altogether.

6. *Bone minerals.* Prepare bone broth soups or consider supplements to support bones.

7. *Inflammation.* Reduce inflammatory foods generally during the fourth trimester.

▮ Bone Loss in Pregnancy and Lactation

A woman will experience some short-term bone loss during pregnancy and breastfeeding. While findings from studies are mixed about what impact this really has on a woman's health in the long term, the bone loss is generally recovered after pregnancy and lactation within a year or so.[9] The increased need of bone mineral metabolism in pregnancy and lactation is clear. Nutritionally supporting this can only be beneficial for both mother and baby in a time of increased need. Perhaps the old wives' tale that said "for every baby, a woman loses a tooth" came about from bone loss during pregnancy and lactation. In our more modern lives, women don't necessarily suffer from malnutrition, thereby decreasing the possibility of losing teeth. In any case, I like to make sure my postpartum women are supplementing with bone minerals either through diet or supplementation. Foods such as bone broth, vegetables, and proteins that are higher in bone minerals and promote metabolic processes (calcium, protein, magnesium, phosphorus, vitamin D, potassium, and fluoride manganese, copper, boron, iron, zinc, vitamin A, vitamin K,

---

9 Salari, P., & Abdollahi, M. (2014). The influence of pregnancy and lactation on maternal bone health: a systematic review. *Journal of Family & Reproductive Health, 8*(4), 135–148.

vitamin C, and the B vitamins) can be a focus during pregnancy and lactation.[10]

Bone Broth Soup Recipe

Bone broth soup is very nourishing after childbirth and gives needed nutrients for healing and breastfeeding support. You can make it in advance and freeze it. Bone broth can then be eaten by itself or as a stock to make other soups. There are a lot of great recipes online. You can also purchase organic bone broth from grocery stores. However, if you like to make your own, below is a general recipe to give you an idea of what bone broth soup is all about.[11]

Choose the following bones:

These types of animal bones are the most warming.

- Beef or lamb (especially good to rebuild blood after blood loss to recover your energy)
- Chicken (especially good to aid a weaker digestion and give you energy)

Choose any of the following vegetables:

These vegetables support the kidney, liver, blood, energy, and enhance immunity.

- Carrots
- Squash

---

10 Palacios, C. (2006). The role of nutrients in bone health, from A to Z, *Critical Reviews in Food Science and Nutrition*, 46(8), 621–628. doi: 10.1080/10408390500466174.

11 Adapted from *7 Times a Woman: Ancient Wisdom on Health & Beauty for Every Stage of Your Life* by Dr. Lia Andrews.

- Beets
- Celery
- Leeks
- Dark greens like collards
- Parsley

Choose any of the following spices:

These spices are warming, support electrolyte balance, and enhance immunity.

- Ginger
- Cinnamon
- Cardamom
- Clove
- Turmeric
- Fennel
- Pepper
- Good salt

Directions:

1. Rinse about 5 pounds of bones to remove any dirt or blood.
2. Roast the bones in the oven at 425 degrees Fahrenheit for 1–2 hours to enhance flavor.
3. Bring 5 quarts of cold water to boil and then bring it down to a simmer.
4. Add bones.
5. Skim bubbles and scum until water is clear.
6. Add the spices you prefer and to taste, then simmer for 4–5 hours.
7. Add 2 ½ cups of vegetables and cook for another 1–2 hours.
8. Strain all the vegetables and bones.
9. Use stock within a few days or freeze stock for future use.

Inflammatory Foods Affecting Healing and Breastfeeding

Some foods may cause physical inflammation in your digestive system, which is disruptive to a healthy digestive process. This in turn may affect your breast milk and cause your baby's digestion to be very reactive (gas, bloating, colic, reflux, or frequent spitting up). If this is happening, look through the following list of foods and adjust your diet.

As much as keeping a warm digestion is important, some foods fall into an inflammatory category because they are hot or produce heat toxins in the body. If you are not sensitive to inflammation, you may have less trouble with these foods. But if you tend to have food sensitivities, you may have more severe reactions or it can pass on to your baby whilst breastfeeding.

Below is a list of the common inflammatory food groups and some examples of how you can apply the warm digestion concept (where appropriate) to reduce the effect of that inflammatory food in your diet. Perhaps you don't need to completely eliminate these foods during the postpartum period or during breastfeeding. As your baby grows, their digestion will begin to mature as well. Foods that may affect them more in the first month may not affect them as much by the fourth month, for example.

Gluten. This includes wheat, rye, oats, and barley, which are commonly found in breads, pasta, and other products made with refined flour. Gluten is a very common allergy and inflammatory substance. Studies are still unclear as to whether it's gluten itself or some component of the grain brought out either through growth or production that causes an allergic reaction.

- <u>Warm Digestion Concept:</u> Sprouted grains, such as bread made from sprouted wheat, can reduce the inflammation and sensitivity in the digestion.

Highly processed forms of gluten often cause more inflammation and irritation.

Alcohol and Caffeine. Both alcohol and caffeine can affect the functioning of the liver, kidneys, and blood sugar regulation systems and have other long-term health and inflammation repercussions. It's best to avoid caffeine in any amount, since it acts as a diuretic and can reduce your breast milk volume. Soda, especially diet soda, and processed fruit drinks that are high in simple and refined sugars are hard on the mechanisms that regulate your blood sugar levels. High intakes of sugars, especially synthetic sugars, have been associated with inflammation.

- <u>Warm Digestion Concept:</u> Studies have shown the benefits of moderate use of certain types of alcohol. Red wine, for instance, is warming and is used in preparations of certain Chinese herb formulas to reduce pain and provides other health benefits. For postpartum patients, there is a formula where you cook the herbs in sake (rice wine) and drink this formula for the first month after childbirth. Traditional Chinese Medicine considers even water too cooling for this time in a woman's life.

Meat and Fish. Pork, cold cuts, bacon, hot dogs, canned meats, sausage, and shellfish, as well as meats that are not organic or naturally raised and processed, can be high in hormones, antibiotics, and other undesired ingredients utilized during processing.

- <u>Warm Digestion Concept:</u> Eat natural forms of meats without nitrates or additives, since they will be less reactive.

Eggs and Dairy. All types of milk, cheese, butter, and yogurt produce dampness and phlegm in the body.

- <u>Warm Digestion Concept:</u> Eat farm fresh eggs and harder, drier cheeses. Hormone-free milk, yogurt, and butter can be less reactive.

Vegetables. Corn, tomato sauce, and nightshade vegetables commonly cause inflammation and allergic responses.

- <u>Warm Digestion Concept:</u> Eat more heritage strains grown without pesticides, and eat them when they're in season.

Fruit. Citrus fruits, juices, strawberries, and pineapples are common allergens or produce phlegm. They also produce a cooling effect to the digestion and may adversely affect blood sugar regulation.

- <u>Warm Digestion Concept:</u> Cooking fruit can have a warming affect; however, if your baby is having a reaction when you eat fruit whether or not it is cooked, it is best to avoid fruit altogether until your baby is older.

Fat. Foods high in saturated fats and refined oils, such as peanuts, margarine, and shortening, may be inflammatory, as processing these foods places an extra burden on the system.

- <u>Warm Digestion Concept:</u> Less processed, good oils and fats have a true health benefit in the body's systems.

Other common foods that may affect breast milk include:

- chocolate

- spices, such as cinnamon, garlic, curry, chili pepper

- citrus fruits and their juices, like oranges, lemons, limes, and grapefruits

- fruits with a laxative effect, such as cherries and prunes

- other fruits that act as common allergens, such as strawberries, kiwis, and pineapples

- the "gassy" veggies, such as onion, cabbage, garlic, cauliflower, broccoli, cucumbers, and peppers

SUMMARY: WHAT TO BUY AND PREPARE BEFORE GIVING BIRTH

■ 1. PREPARE YOUR POSTPARTUM PANTRY

You can always follow the warm digestion guidelines above. Cook and freeze food in advance.

A beautiful book called *The First Forty Days: The Essential Art of Nourishing the New Mother* by Heng Ou goes into depth about all the foods, incredible recipes, and how to put together your postpartum pantry from an Asian perspective.

■ 2. PREPARE YOUR POSTPARTUM HEALING KIT

- Abdominal wrap for postpartum healing
- Perineal spray bottle
- Sitz baths
- Nipple cream (if breastfeeding)
- Belly oil or cream
- Postpartum herbal formula (consult with a licensed acupuncturist or Chinese Medicine practitioner for this)
- Post-pregnancy panties

- Overnight menstrual pads for postpartum bleeding
- Witch hazel pads for vaginal births

▰ 3. MAKE YOUR POSTPARTUM PLAN

Make a plan to optimize resting and healing, especially in the first month, based on the principles of this book.

Reach out for help and resources before you give birth, such as specialists, to understand how they can help and support you and your baby.

IN CLOSING:
A NEW BEGINNING

I'm writing the closing to this book seven weeks into my region's quarantine during the COVID-19 global pandemic. For six weeks, this book sat untouched, even though it was so close to being finished. I was occupied with transitioning my patients to telehealth, learning about COVID-19, and trying to maintain continuity of care with an abrupt halt without warning. It has been a life-changing event for me, as I am sure it has been for many of you. So many things going forward from this moment will change. Hopefully we, as a collective, take this opportunity to consider other ways we might approach health in general and, more specifically, how we approach postpartum care. Let's use all the tools from all credible health approaches to achieve better outcomes. My hope is that this book serves as one of those useful tools to add to your postpartum toolbox.

The pandemic was unexpected, to say the least, but there are some silver linings that have directly affected my approach to postpartum care. Most important is the power of telehealth. This revelation has led me to recommit resources and access for my patients' continuity of care. I had to think outside of the box in order to deliver health care in a whole new way with virtual acupuncture sessions, which offer a dynamic, relevant mode of care that can now be utilized postpartum in the safety of your own home. I hope this novel addition to health care, plus other developments such as the accessibility of food and grocery delivery, lead to the adoption of a "resting month" among more and more new mothers.

Lastly, I encourage you to check out the online resources section on my website at TansyBriggs.com and take a look at the growing collaboration with online resources to support postpartum moms. Rather than a closing to this book, this is more like a new beginning. I wish you a healthy postpartum as you prepare, recover, nourish and heal.

Yours in health,
Tansy Briggs, DACM

APPENDIX:

Key nutrients and foods

Folic Acid/ Folate	• up to 400–800mcg/day including supplemental sources • green leafy veggies, root veggies, whole grains, wheat germ, nuts, milk, salmon
Iron	• molasses, whole grains, wheat germ, red meat, poultry, egg yolk, avocados, almonds, dried figs, currants, green leafy veggies
Vitamin A	• egg yolk, butter, cheese, yogurt, carrots, spinach, broccoli, apples, mangoes
Vitamin B	• egg yolk, molasses, whole grains, wheat germ, rice, legumes, green veggies, bananas, papayas, dried peaches, prunes
Vitamin C	• citrus fruits (avoid oranges and orange juice), black currants, melons, pineapples, bananas, raspberries, apples, prunes, tomatoes, potatoes, brussels sprouts, kale, broccoli, parsley, alfalfa, rose hips
Vitamin E	• unrefined, cold pressed oils (like olive or flax), whole grains, wheat germ, nuts, green leafy veggies, avocados, molasses, eggs
Zinc	• meat, poultry, fish, ginger, sunflower, sesame, pumpkin seeds, sprouted seeds, almonds, soybeans, green leafy veggies, watercress, wheat germ, oat germ, whole grains
Calcium	• whole grains, nuts, dairy products, carob, dolomite, green leafy veggies
Chromium	• molasses, whole grains, wheat germ, veggies, butter
Essential Fatty Acids	• nuts, unrefined oils, nut butters (almond, sesame), green leafy veggies, seeds (sunflower), oily fish (mackerel, tuna)
Magnesium	• nuts, kelp, seafood, eggs, milk, whole grains, green veggies, dolomite
Selenium	• tuna, herring, butter, wheat germ, brazil nuts, garlic, whole grains
Vitamin D	• whole milk, cheese, yogurt, eggs, fish oil, fatty fish
Vitamin K	• cauliflower, cabbage, egg yolks, green leafy veggies, soybeans

Appendix

Nutrient needs through the trimesters

First Trimester

Folic Acid/Folate: (up to 400ug/day including supplement sources) green leafy veggies, root veggies, whole grains, wheat germ, milk, salmon, nuts
Iron: molasses, whole grains, wheat germ, red meat, poultry, egg yolk, almonds, dried figs, currants, avocados, green leafy veggies
Vitamin A: egg yolk, butter, cheese, yogurt, carrots, spinach, broccoli, apples, mangoes
Vitamin B: egg yolk, molasses, whole grains, wheat germ, rice, legumes, green veggies, bananas, papayas, dried peaches, prunes
Vitamin C: citrus fruits (avoid oranges and orange juice), black currants, melons, pineapples, bananas, raspberries, apples, prunes, tomatoes, potatoes, brussels sprouts, kale, broccoli, parsley, alfalfa, rose hips
Vitamin E: unrefined, cold pressed oils (like olive or flax) whole grains, wheat germ, nuts, green leafy veggies, avocados, molasses, and eggs
Zinc: meat, poultry, fish, ginger, sunflower seeds, sesame seeds, pumpkin seeds, sprouted seeds, almonds, soybeans, green leafy veggies, watercress, wheat germ, oat germ, whole grains

Second Trimester

Calcium: whole grains, nuts, dairy products, carob, dolomite, green leafy veggies
Chromium: molasses, whole grains, wheat germ, veggies, butter
Essential Fatty Acids: nuts, unrefined oils, nut butters (almond, sesame, etc.), green leafy veggies, seeds (sunflower), oily fish (mackerel, tuna)
Magnesium: nuts, kelp, seafood, eggs, milk, whole grains, green veggies, dolomite
Selenium: tuna, herring, butter, wheat germ, brazil nuts, garlic, whole grains
Vitamin D: whole milk, cheese, yogurt, eggs, fish oil, fatty fish

Third Trimester

Vitamin K: cauliflower, cabbage, egg yolks, green leafy veggies, soybeans

Nutrients Through the Trimesters

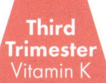

Third Trimester
Vitamin K

Second Trimester
Calcium
Chromium
Essential Fatty Acids
Magnesium
Selenium
Vitamin D

First Trimester
Folic Acid/Folate
Iron
Zinc
Vitamins A, B, C, E

List of foods and corresponding temperatures

Neutral	Warm	Hot
Fruits apricot, loquat, papaya, pomegranate, tangerine, peaches, lemon	**Fruits** blackberry, cherry, dates, grape, litchi, longan, quince, raspberry, strawberry*, kumquat, figs	**Fruits** pineapple*
Vegetables beets, carrot, cabbage, lettuce, shitake mushroom, olive, peas, pumpkin, yam	**Vegetables** bell peppers*, chive, green bean, kale, leek, mustard greens, parsley, parsnip, squash, sweet potato, watercress, scallions, onion, fennel, oyster mushroom	**Vegetables** garlic, green onion
Grains, Legumes & Nuts brown rice, corn, flax, white rice, almonds, chickpeas, hazelnut, peanut, pistachio, pumpkin, sunflower seeds	**Grains, Legumes & Nuts** oats, quinoa, safflower, spelt, black bean, chestnut, pine nut, sesame seed, walnut	**Animal Products** lamb, trout
Animal Products abalone, rabbit, cheese, duck, goose, herring, mackerel, milk, oysters, salmon, sardine, shark, tuna, chicken	**Animal Products** beef, liver, anchovy, butter, chicken, eel, ham, lobster, mussels, shrimp, turkey, venison, fresh-water fish, sheep, goat, sheep milk	**Spices & Oils** black pepper, cayenne pepper, chili pepper, cinnamon, dry ginger, horseradish, wasabi, mustard, garlic
Spices & Oils coriander, licorice, saffron, olive oil, peanut oil	**Spices & Oils** anise, basil, bay leaf, carob, caraway, clove, cumin, dill seed, fennel, fenugreek, fresh ginger, nutmeg, oregano, rosemary, sage, spearmint, thyme, jasmine, coriander	*indicates potentially inflammatory food*

RESOURCES

▪ Online:

TansyBriggs.com

▪ Books:

Postpartum Support

7 Times a Woman: Ancient Wisdom on Health and Beauty for Every Stage of Your Life by Lia Andrews

Balance Your Hormones, Balance Your Life by Claudia Welch

The First Forty Days: The Essential Art of Nourishing the Mother by Heng Ou, Amely Greeven, and Marisa Belger

The Key to a Healthy Digestion: How to Eat Warm and Cold Foods to Improve Your Health by Tansy Briggs

Working Mothers Support

The Fifth Trimester: The Working Mom's Guide to Style, Sanity, and Big Success After Baby by Lauren Smith Brody

For Practitioners and Health Care Providers

Acupressure and Acupuncture During Birth by Claudia Citkovitz

Acupuncture in Pregnancy and Childbirth by Zita West

The Essential Guide to Acupuncture in Pregnancy and Childbirth by Debra Betts

CPSIA information can be obtained
at www.ICGtesting.com
Printed in the USA
LVHW070740140920
665931LV00008B/148